Fitness Lifestyle For The Career Professional

Table of Contents

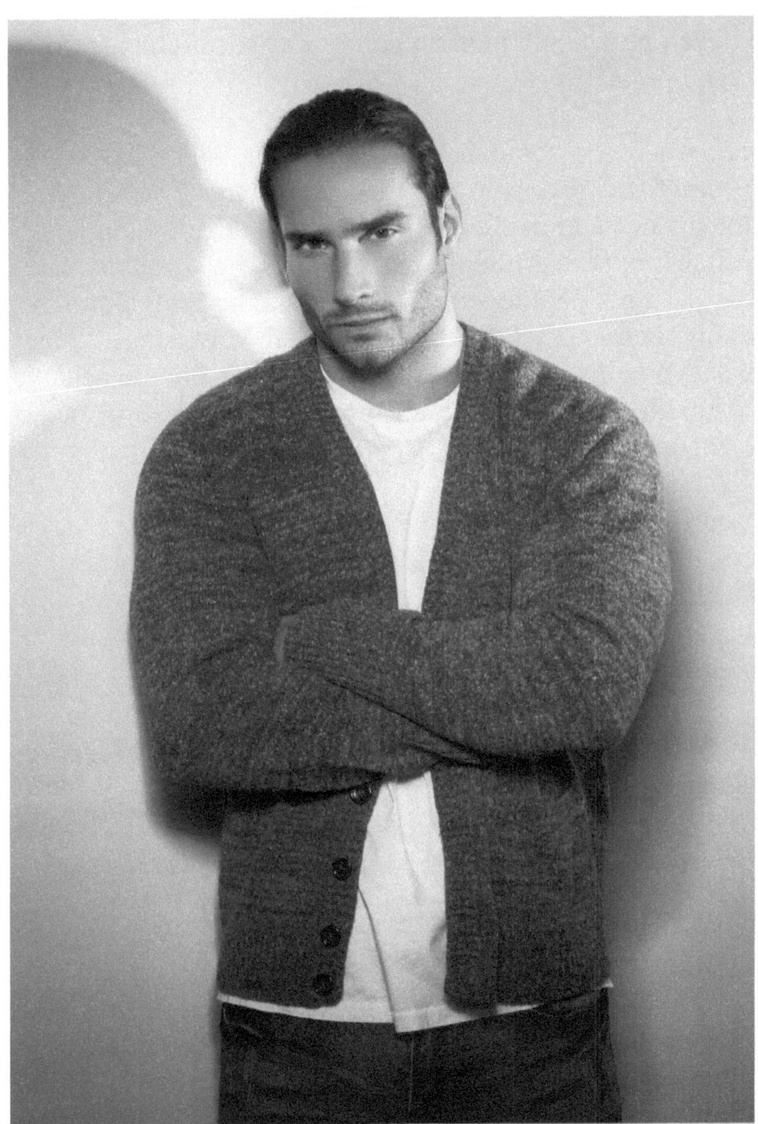

Eugene Dinescu is one of the world's leading health and wellness experts, specializing in metabolism. He is a world-renowned biochemist from Columbia University with publications in metabolic pathways and is hired as a health and wellness speaker, consultant, and educator throughout the United States. He created a first-of-kind Health and Wellness Initiative that is now being implemented in New Jersey State Approved Private Schools. The first school to adopt Eugene's program Westbridge Academy, is currently in its 10th year, and has saved New Jersey State an estimated $4.5M. His company, The Potential Group, works with schools around the state of New Jersey to satisfy New Jersey Department of Education professional development and nutrition programs requirements in statute, code, and regulations.

Growing up, he was a star football, track and field, and soccer athlete. His desire to achieve peak physical performance combined with a love for science and medicine makes him a one of a kind health and wellness expert. Although just hobbies, he was able to achieve success as a national level powerlifter and bodybuilder. One of the keys to his success: diet. Eugene lives by the old adage, "you are what you eat" and his goal is to educate others on how to achieve their personal health and wellness goals through proper eating and accurate information.

There's a lot of misinformation when it comes to dieting and Eugene wants to dispel the common myths and make things simple and straightforward for everyone. With over 20 years of experience, proven results, and unparalleled knowledge, there is no one better to teach you about how you should be eating.

If you want to know when Eugene's next book will come out, please visit his website at http://www.eugenedinescu.com, where you can sign up to receive an email when he has his next release.

Why did I write this book?

I wrote this book for two main reasons. Firstly, there isn't any fitness book out there that caters to professional people. This has always boggled my mind. You see all of these famous fitness personalities on the web, Instagram, YouTube, Facebook, etc., however most of these people don't have real jobs or careers like you or me. In fact, most don't even really work nor have they ever held a professional career job within a demanding industry. Therefore, how can they understand how to educate you on living a healthy fitness oriented lifestyle? They simply can't. Fortunately for you, I'm just like you. If you read my biography on the front page I don't have to reiterate my life story. You know that I have been super busy most of my life yet I've been able to stay in great shape throughout my career. How was I able to accomplish this? Well, I'm going to show you.

The second reason I wrote this book is the most important reason: I want to help you. I genuinely believe in giving back. I'm highly accomplished in my career and truthfully writing is just a hobby for me. Whether or not this book becomes a top seller or is used as a coffee cup mat is all up to the Universe. It would be nice to have a book that is well received by many however I can't control that outcome. I can only do my best just like you. I truly hope that you find great utility in this book.

With that said, I want to mention a few things upfront. I chose to write this book as if you and I are sitting down talking over a beer or glass of wine. Beer and wine? I thought this book was all about a fitness lifestyle. Yes, of course it is. However, you want to have a life too? Don't ya? As a professional I'm always going to social events and there's nothing wrong in my book (did you catch that pun?) with having a drink or two. Everything in moderation as the old adage said eons ago. In fact, I'm a firm believer that being too rigid will likely do more harm than good. I learned this from personal experience. There was a time when I was so strict with everything that I did that I was constantly stressed out. The key is to just chill out and have a relaxed demeanor while sticking to your priorities. I'm not condoning eating like crap all of the time or binge drinking. I'm just saying that we are all just mere humans and let's enjoy this life to the fullest.

You will never stick to anything that you hate. I'm well aware of this. Therefore, my job in this book will be to show you how you can enjoy the best of both worlds. Flourish in your career as well as live a healthy fit lifestyle. If you're wondering where the career chapters of this book are located then it means you purchased the discounted version of this book and I must say you get what you pay for. Just kidding, the success within your career is one hundred percent all you for now. I'll have other books in the future on topics like that. All I can promise here is that I will show you exactly how you can also maximize your health and fitness in conjunction with any career.

The last thing that I want to say is please don't expect this to be easy. Come on, we are both career people, we both know that nothing worth anything of real value in this world is easily attainable, right? Thus, obviously, juggling your career, eating healthy, and going to the gym is not going to be easy. Don't let that deter you. The good news is that I'm going to make it as "relatively" easy as possible. I'm going to make it realistic for you unlike all of these fitness gurus that have never held a real job in their lives.

Why this book will change your life?

By the laws of basic deduction if you purchased this book chances are that you are a professional career person and that you feel that you have room for improvement regarding your fitness lifestyle. I personally believe there's always room for improvement as I'm constantly improving myself. Maybe you have a nonexistent fitness routine and you don't follow a healthy diet. No matter what part of the spectrum you fall under this book will one hundred percent help you in some way. It will give you answers that you have been looking for, not all of them, because I don't think any one person possesses all of the answers. Remember when we would take standardized tests and we were told, never choose the extreme answer choices, well, that's because extreme anything doesn't work and someone that tell you that they know everything probably does not. This book will give you a lot of answers. Not only did I try to make it entertaining to read and unique, but it will also be jam packed with information that I personally have never seen anywhere else.

If you have purchased other books that I have written you know that I don't like wasting time. I also don't really follow standard rules and conventions, especially in writing; I think that's boring and unoriginal. I think being different is cool. I think being good is good. I think being different and good is great. I believe in thinking outside of the box and I question everything. Therefore, I think that you should also question me as well as all of the information out there. I encourage you to constantly ask why did he write that or why did he include that? There should be a purpose as I mentioned before I don't like wasting time. As a businessman and serial entrepreneur, I need to understand the bottom line and I need to understand it as quickly as possible. And I'm fully expecting that you do as well.

Thus, I'm going to conclude this chapter soon. Before I do so. I'm going to make several assumptions that directly relate to how this book will change your life.

Assumption number one: you are very busy and you believe that there is absolutely no way that you can maintain a high level career as well as an exceptional physique because doing both is just unrealistic.

Assumption number two: you hear and read tons of conflicting information about the best diets but you just don't know what to believe.

Assumption number three: you hear and read tons of conflicting information about the best exercise routines but you don't know what to believe.

Assumption number four: you don't even want to begin anything because you believe that it is likely going to fail or it is just some other fad.

Assumption number five: you purchased this book because you are looking for hope and somewhere or somehow you heard of me, the guy who tells it like it is and has built a reputation of honesty and integrity, and you thought, you never know, let's give this a shot.

If any or all of my assumptions are correct, I will tell you that you are in luck. I will show you that you are not too busy, I will teach you how to eat, I will teach you how to exercise effectively, and I will show you why I have built the reputation that I have.

The moment that you adopt my strategies for embracing a fitness lifestyle your life will dramatically change. You will feel better, you will be happier, you will look better naked (which is always a plus), you will be healthier, and you will live a higher quality life. I will tell you this, nothing in the world compares to living a healthy lifestyle. I have experienced most things in life material as well as experiential and nothing compares to being the best version of yourself: in mind, body, and spirit.

How to get started

Okay, you decided that's it. You're motivated and inspired. It's time you make changes. If this guy Eugene can actually take into account my super busy schedule and somehow teach me how to also live a fitness lifestyle, I'm sold. Let's go. The first thing you need to do is focus on your mind. The same way that you decided you're going to be successful in your career and you're going to do whatever it takes to realize your goals in your career, you're going to apply that same mindset to you body and health. You will accomplish nothing without a strong mind. You know this. Therefore, let's go through some mental exercises combined with some simple conditioning to get you ready and then get you on your way to fitness success.

This is going to sound really funny but I recommend watching motivational YouTube videos. There's just so much good content out there and it doesn't need to be fitness related. You just need to prime your mind for something new. This is going to be a new undertaking and trust me when I tell you; you're going to need all of the tools you can get to ensure that you really do succeed, not just for the short term, but also for the long term. I literally watch something motivational every single day. That's how I get fired up. Use my trick. Try it out. Right now you're not working out. You're not eating healthy. But watch something that really resonates deep within you and I bet you're going to want to get up and go do something. For the sake of this book, that something should be eating healthy and working out.

The second trick that I encourage you to do is read some inspirational quotes from people that you admire. Again this takes only a few seconds but has lasting effects. As you can see, I try to immerse my mind with positive thoughts and affirmations. You must do the same. Now you have just activated most of your senses and this will have positive effects on your mentality. Neurobiological research has shown us that through eliciting multiple senses simultaneously stronger emotions and memories will persist. If you want almost every sense to be activated why don't you light a candle and chew your favorite flavor of gym while you're reading this? I'm just kidding, did you actually take me seriously? On a serious note, if you do have candles make sure that they are soy candles as the other types are toxic and don't chew gum. I have never found gum that does not contain at least one harmful chemical such as titanium dioxide. Metals like that interfere with your brain and cognitive abilities. Unfortunately, I don't think there is any healthy gum out there. This is just my recommendation. Just brush your teeth after you eat and you should be fine.

The third trick that you should employ is eliminating anything negative from your life. Life is hard as it is. You can't have negative elements in your life and expect to be your best self. Especially when embarking on something difficult. Therefore, if you are in a toxic relationship, I recommend you let it go. After you follow my plan for a few months you'll do much better anyway. If you have friends that are negative influences around you, try to minimize the time you spend with them. If you engage in unhealthy bad habits such as excessive partying, drinking, or drug use, you need to stop all of that. There's nothing wrong with partying and anyone that knows me knows that I love a good party however drugs are a no go for me and they should be for you. If I were a stronger man I would give up my social drinking as well. Unfortunately, the key word is "if" and I'm just not that strong. Nobody is perfect. Accept that. However, we should recognize our flaws and try to do better. Also, as I mentioned before, I subscribe to balance. I think as long as you maintain a healthy balance you should be fine. If you did not know excessive drinking can destroy your liver and you can develop something called liver cirrhosis – basically chronic liver damage leading to scarring and liver failure.

The fourth and final trick that I think you should use during this process is to visualize your ideal self. Think about who you would want to be. I'm not saying you're not good enough. I'm sure you are. I'm just saying that we all have room for improvement. Nobody is perfect. Moreover, due to the second law of thermodynamics we are actually in a constant state of decay via entropy. On a positive note, healthy eating combined with exercise has been shown to reverse signs of aging. I strategically placed the word "signs" in the last sentence because I've heard nonsense that goes something like this: "you can reverse aging." No, that is scientifically impossible according to the laws of nature. What you can do is you can reduce the rate at which you age and you can also eliminate certain signs of aging giving off the appearance of age reversal. What are some quick signs? Hair, skin, and nails are all indicators of health for most people. Unless you suffer from an autoimmune disorder like psoriasis your hair, skin, and nails can certainly be looked at as representative of how well you take care of yourself. I would like to mention that through healthy eating and exercising, autoimmune disorders could be greatly nullified. According to all of the research, autoimmune disorders are on a consistent rise. I believe that this is due mostly to our diets and sedentary lifestyles but that's just my opinion.

Okay, so now you know some of my tricks for success. I say that these are tricks for success in general because they are applicable to any goal that you may have. For you, I want you to focus and zone in on your food intake and exercise plan. We still have a bit more to discuss. If you want to skip to the diet and exercise plan of this book feel free to do so however I think that the next couple of chapters will add value to your life. Otherwise I would have just written a book with two chapters: diet and exercise.

Before beginning the diet and exercise routine that I have here I want you to slowly adapt yourself and plan for when you will exercise. For instance, if you work a standard nine to five, you need to make a decision. Will you work out before work or will you work out after work? I will tell you that it doesn't matter what time of day you workout. That is a really stupid myth. People try to track levels of hormone production and come up with ideal workout times. For instance, some research I've seen indicates that testosterone peaks during early afternoon and for that reason, it's best to workout at that time. If you have the mindset that you need to depend on when you're testosterone levels are peaking in order to get into the gym, then you need to go back to my tricks one through four and repeat them. Your will is unbreakable and no matter what you will achieve your goals. That's the mindset you must have if you want to succeed here. Who cares if you testosterone is in flux? Everything in life is in flux. I've said this before, but life is just one long sine wave, the sine wave from calculus, yes I'm nerdy, you're probably nerdy too.

Okay, so have you decided what time of day you will workout? Good. Now you need to adjust your schedule accordingly to get used to what you're about to do. There's no need for you to look at the exercise routine right now. We are taking baby steps. What I want you to do is begin going to the gym now. I recommend doing cardio or taking a yoga class that fits within the schedule you just set up. Start out by going just twice a week. You can choose the days. Increase by one day every week or two until you are now going to the gym five days a week. If you can do this you will basically have half of the battle won when it comes to exercising. Be patient with yourself. However, don't make excuses. Excuses only get you more excuses. In all of my life, I have almost never missed a workout no matter what. Even if I was on a business trip and just got off of a flight without sleeping for over twenty hours or so, I would still make it to the gym. I just modify my workout so that I don't hurt myself and that's what you need to learn to do. This brings me to the next chapter.

A consistent but flexible schedule

You must be consistent. You must be flexible. Have you noticed that nobody in health and fitness ever talks about having a flexible mindset? They're just so extreme, "you have to do this and you have do it this way and you have to do it at this specific time." This entire process should be fun. Eating healthy should be fun. Working out should be fun. My approach is a serious approach but I believe you need to be consistent but not too rigid. What do I mean by this?

As I mentioned in the previous chapter, you must workout on all of your committed days. That's a must. However, you can adapt to your schedule or to things that may pop up. If you're a professional, you will always have something. Therefore you need to get used to being flexible. I told you to build the habit of going to the gym up until you achieve five days a week. In the beginning believe it or not, you need to be more rigid than after it becomes your life. I never have a set schedule for my eating or my exercising. I just consistently eat three to four healthy meals a day and I consistently exercise once a day five to six days a week. Even my workouts are flexible. Some days I feel better than others. Some days I feel worse. You need to be flexible and adaptable.

Being flexible will unlock something very valuable for you. With a flexible mindset, you will no longer put pressure on yourself. You will actually learn to have fun doing all of these things. Let me give you an example. Let's imagine a realistic scenario. You have committed to working out every afternoon after work around six in the evening. Unfortunately, your boss tells you that you need to attend an event from six to eight on Tuesday. Tuesday is one of your workout days and six to eight is when you workout. If you don't have a flexible mindset, you're going to feel stressed and you're going to likely panic when it comes to juggling your career responsibilities with your exercise responsibilities. Repeated events like this will disrupt your health and fitness goals. Here are three solutions that I use myself:

Solution one: I don't stress. I workout after the event. I'll just get less sleep. In my mind I condition myself to think of the situation as no big deal. I'll adjust my workout to be easier and shorter than normal. The fitness lifestyle is for life, not a week. Therefore, I can always just train harder next week.

Solution two: I don't stress. I workout before work since I have a heads up on the event. I can probably plan accordingly and not even compromise my sleep. I will have to make some modifications as in bring my work stuff with me and shower at the gym but so what. Again, problem solved with ease.

Solution three: I don't stress. I combine the workout that I was supposed to do on Tuesday with Wednesday's workout. Again, you never stress with these things.

You choose which solution works for you. You're going to need to think outside of the box often when juggling multiple difficult things at a time. You're aware of this. However, I'm just demonstrating to you how easily you can solve a fitness-career related issue. Let's assume you have another scenario such as a business trip for an entire week or two in another country. This is something I have to deal with often. It's not that big of a deal. Most countries have gyms. If you can't find a gym you can improvise. I will discuss improvising later.

Habits

I'm sure you understand the value of good habits. Habits are so vital for your success that you must actively try to develop and instill good habits. We have discussed a lot so far. This chapter is incredibly important. Your habits when it comes to eating healthily and exercising consistently can make or break whether or not you will be successful long term. It's all up to you to start out on the right foot and maintain good habits.

What do I mean? Simply put, if you want to seriously achieve the best version of yourself you're going to need to cook your food or you're going to need to have someone, like a personal chef, cook your food. Let's assume that you don't have a personal chef at your disposal. If you are in that situation, you will have to form the habit of cooking consistently for yourself. The task of home cooking can be daunting for anyone who has never done this before. However, it is easy to learn how to cook. I will discuss it more in depth in the nutrition section of this book but it is really very easy. Cooking healthy food is ironically much easier than cooking unhealthy food because the food will be simple within minimal ingredients. So cooking every two or three days is a habit you must develop.

What other habits should you have? Let's assume you are working out consistently. One of the most important things is to form good workout habits; again, I will discuss this in depth in the exercise section. However, good exercise habits are warming up before beginning, challenging yourself in the gym, and not doing yourself a disservice by underperforming. More than seventy percent of people in the gym from my personal observations are pretty much just wasting their time. Don't become one of these people. Go to the gym with purpose. Good habits will ensure that you are effective.

The efficient workout

How do I efficiently workout? What type of workout should I do? How long should the workout be? Do I need to do cardio? Should I train one body part per day? I'm sure that you have all of these questions and I'm going to break down the answer to each one of these questions.

What is the efficient workout? Okay, so the general answer to this question is the following: the efficient workout is a workout in which you achieve maximum results with minimal time investment. Here's where things get a little tricky. No two people are going to follow the same exact workout plan or exercise regiment. Why? Simply put, we are all different. We have different goals for how we want to look. Additionally, different exercises are better for different people. I know you were looking for a cookie cutter explanation of the efficient workout. I'm sorry but I'm not in the business of providing you with cookie cutter exercise plans. Fortunately, as you will see later on the diet is a little bit different since virtually all people should follow certain rules when it comes to nutrition.

Okay, so back to the efficient workout or exercise regiment. The most important thing that you need to do is to decide your goals. How do you want to look? How do you want to perform? Are you exercising strictly for health related reasons? You must answer all of these questions. Once you have a solid vision then you can craft a logical workout routine.

In order to provide you with a real life example I'm going to tell you about what I do. Keep in mind that you may not have my goals. After I give you my workout regiment I'm going to give you the rationale behind every element. With this knowledge it is my hope that you will be able to develop a logical routine that fits your goals. Don't just imitate other people and don't get conditioned to just follow exactly what you're told. What if there's a better way? Try to learn from everyone.

I make sure that every workout does not take more than two hours at the longest. I also make sure that I incorporate at least four to five muscle groups per workout. Lastly, I make sure that I always do cardio after every weight training session.

Two hours may seem like a long time however for my specific goals it is what I require some of the time. Some of my workouts are only one hour in duration. I train several body parts during each workout because I found that to work best for my body and I also don't want to gain any more muscle. I prefer to stay as lean as I can and training four to five body parts allows me to maintain a relatively low body fat. I also do cardio after every workout because cardio is one hundred percent essential for optimal results and my cardio is intense so I get a leg workout every day to some degree. If you are trying to put on muscle and you have subscribed to the notion that cardio will zap you of your muscle mass, you could not be any further from the truth. Of course, excessive cardio in the wrong form can hurt your muscle gaining goals. However, just the right amount will only enhance your ability to put on and maintain muscle. Remember that weight training does not effectively work your heart as well as other organs like your lungs. You need to do cardio to work your heart. The strength of your heart is directly correlated to your heart's ability to pump blood throughout your body. The only way that nutrients are delivered throughout your body is through your circulation. Thus, I think you now understand why it is vital for you to do cardio.

Let's go through some rules that I have to make sure that my workouts are maximally efficient:

Rule number one: no socializing. The gym is not social hour. There's nothing wrong with greeting your friends at the gym however having full blown conversations will zap your time and destroy efficiency. I always say hi to my friends at the gym.

Rule number two: no gym partners. I choose not to have a gym partner because you don't want to be dependent on another person. We are all busy and we all have our own lives. What happens if your gym partner can't make it? Are you not going to go to the gym? Are you going to have a lower quality workout? This can't be an option. In rare cases, if you feel that a gym partner is adding value to your exercise plan then I encourage it. However, in most instances, I think it's best to get in to the habit of going solo.

Rule number three: minimal rest in between sets. I personally only do three to four sets per exercise and I do not rest more than a minute. Large rest breaks will destroy efficiency.

Rule number four: listen to music. Listening to some of your favorite tracks can serve as positive reinforcement when you're in the gym exercising with weights or doing cardio. Unless you really don't enjoy listening to music I think listening to great music can certainly put you in the mood and help you stay there.

Rule number five: no lingering around after the workout. Once my workout is done, I'm straight to the locker room and then out of the door. I don't hangout.

Those are my general rules for making sure that I'm always efficient. I think that if you follow these rules you will waste minimal time in the gym.

If you are really curious to know what my entire workout looks like here is where it currently stands as of 2018. I believe in adding value and maybe you will adopt this workout for your own.

My exercise regiment always begins on Sunday. Sunday I train legs, back, and abdominals. I choose to begin on Sunday because Monday is the beginning of the workweek and I like to mentally get myself prepared for work (although truthfully I work seven days a week). By going to the gym Sunday I feel that I have already prepared myself for the week and I already started to put effort into something. It's a good warm up as you may say for the demanding week. Additionally, I choose to train legs on the first day of my exercise regiment because legs are typically neglected and in my personal opinion the least enjoyable to train. However, that's just me. Perhaps you may love training legs. Everyone is different.

How does my workout go? I start my leg workout by doing three sets of leg extensions with a superset of hamstring curls. If you don't know standard exercise lingo, here is what the above sentence means: basically, I use the leg extension machine and then I immediately use the hamstring curl machine. I do three sets of this. I personally do not take any rest during this part of the workout. After the three sets of leg extensions and hamstring curls I go over to do free weight squats. I do about four to five sets increasing the weight load with each subsequent set. Afterwards I go to leg press and I do four to five sets increasing the weight load. I usually do one leg at a time on the leg press first and then I'll train both legs on the leg press. Next I do stiff legged Romanian deadlifts; no I don't do them because I'm Romanian, LOL. Finally I do one exercise and three sets of that exercise like standing calve raises for calves. After legs, I do about ten sets of pull-ups with a superset of leg raises so that I train my back and my abdominals. I finish the entire workout with 15 minutes of cardio. I like to do my cardio on the cycling bike but you can do it however you like. I make sure that every aspect of my workout is as intense as possible, even the bike.

On Monday I train my chest, shoulders, and triceps. I begin the workout with chest. My brother taught me to always warm up my rotator cuffs so I do a few exercises that warms them up before starting on flat barbell bench press. You can also start with dumbbells but I prefer the barbell. I do about four sets of flat bench, four sets of incline, and four sets of decline. My rest periods are very short so this only takes me about fifteen minutes or so. Next I do three sets of an incline fly movement followed by a flat fly movement. I finish the weight training aspect of my workout with three sets of side laterals, three sets of front raises, both exercises targeting the shoulders, and then I do three sets of triceps rope extensions. I then do cardio, fifteen minutes on the bike.

Tuesday consists of training back, biceps, rear deltoids, the trapezius muscles, abdominals, and calves. I begin the workout with back. I do three sets of weighted pull-ups. Then I go to do bent over rows and do about four sets increasing the weight every set. Afterwards I will do pull downs or pull-ups again. I always do three to four sets per exercise. My repetitions vary but are above six reps most times. Since we are on the subject of working out back, I highly recommend avoiding deadlifts as they are very dangerous and I still have yet to meet one avid workout goer who has done deadlifts for over five or so years without injuring his or her back. Therefore, I don't think it's worth it to even do the exercise. After the second round of pull ups, I do dumbbell rows three sets followed by one arm t bar rows followed by t bar rows. I will do three sets of each exercise. I then go to do three sets of hammer curls for biceps. After this, I will do three sets of any rear deltoid exercise I prefer. Once I am done with rear deltoids I will do three sets of calves followed by three sets of leg raises. After leg raises I will do three sets of rope crunches followed by about three minutes of crunches. I finish off the workout as always with cardio. As you can appreciate by now, cardio is imperative; it's just as important, if not more important than the weight-training component.

Wednesday is dedicated to legs and running. For legs I don't do any heavy lifting. I begin the workout by warming my legs up with three sets of leg extensions with a superset of hamstring curls the same as on Sundays. After this, I will do abductor and adductor, three sets of each as a superset. If you've noticed, I always superset exercises working opposing muscle groups. This ensures that you stay symmetrical and balanced. Muscular imbalances can cause many biomechanical and postural issues. After I do the abductor and adductor, I will go do some exercise that will target my gluteus maximus, yes, the butt. Again, I do this so that I am balanced. My goal has always been to have a balanced body. Next I will begin the cardio and running portion of the workout. I warm up with three sets of box jumps followed by one-legged step ups alternating between left and right. Afterwards I will go over to the treadmill and run for about ten to fifteen minutes. I switch things up every time. Sometimes I'll try to run two to three miles at a fast pace. Other times I will do interval training by walking slowly on the treadmill and then sprinting at the max speed that the treadmill permits. Obviously, the maximum speed doesn't simulate a track however for someone who is busy you can't have it all. After I'm done with the treadmill, I will go over to the bike depending on how I feel or I may just call it a day. This workout usually takes me no longer than one hour.

On Thursday I workout one of my favorite muscle groups: shoulders. I do shoulders, abdominals, and calves on this day. For shoulders I begin by warming up my rotator cuff. Please make sure you do this. As I got older, I have learned to appreciate the importance of a proper warm up. After warming up my rotator cuffs I will go do some type of shoulder press exercise, however I don't do any specific type as I'm pretty flexible here. I do about four sets of shoulder press. Then I will do side laterals, three sets. Afterwards, I will do three sets of rear deltoids followed by three sets of front raises. I finish shoulders with three sets of shoulder shrugs. Next I will do three sets of calves raises followed by three sets of leg raises to begin working out abdominals. After the three sets of leg raises I will do cable crunches followed by normal crunches. I should mention that I do not count reps on any exercise for any body part. Sometimes, I consciously know how many reps I've performed however I believe in intuitive training and just listening to your body. Therefore, to me, it doesn't make sense to count my reps since one day I may be able to do ten reps and another day only eight. It's all about pushing yourself to your max every exercise every set. Sort of how life is. You just give it your all. After I'm done with abdominals I will go and do fifteen minutes of cardio on the bike.

Friday is a fun day since I train almost every muscle group in my body. I guess I should mention that every day is sort of like leg day for me because I push myself extremely hard on the cycling at the end of my workouts. I always bike on a very high gear so that it's difficult to move the pedals. Anyway, let's get back to Friday. I begin the workout by doing a superset of biceps and triceps. I will do four sets of barbell bicep curls with four sets of inside bench for the triceps. This is all a superset. Next I will do dumbbell curls, four sets, with four sets of skull crushers, superset. Don't worry; if you are safe you won't crush your skull. If you have no idea what this exercise is, you can either Google it, or you can just choose something else for triceps. Please don't ever stress working out, it's such an easy thing to do in life. You just need to get to the gym. That's all. Okay, so after dumbbell curls and skull crushers, I will do three sets of hammer curls with three sets of overhead dumbbell extensions superset. I usually do one mega set of as many reps as possible of forearm wrist curls. After this, I begin working out my chest and back. I start out by doing pull ups with a superset of flat bench. I do four sets of this. Next I will do pull-ups with incline bench, again four sets. After this, I may do pulls ups and dips or I may just go to cardio. It all depends on how much time I have and how I feel. As you probably guessed, I will go to do cycling for my cardio, as this is my preferred form of cardio. Even though I'm relatively young, I sort of selected cycling as my go to exercise for cardio because of several reasons. Cycling can be really intense, it is safe, and I think that I can likely do it all of my life without hurting my joints. If you run instead of cycle, you will put some stress on your joints, especially your knees, and as you get older you will likely have to reduce your running or stop running altogether. I tend to think about the future, thus cycling made the most sense.

Saturdays are my designated off day. Saturdays also happen to be my fun day for the week. If for whatever reason I have not done some fun activity that week or social event I will likely do something of that nature on Saturday. Not all the time though. Some Saturdays are dedicated to more work, reading, and writing. Being an entrepreneur, I work so many hours every day that there's never enough time. A nine to five doesn't exist for me. Anyway, Saturdays are usually fun days. Now let's get into the theory behind training multiple muscle groups.

Why train multiple muscle groups?

I personally have come to deduce several theories that I believe to be true for most humans. Firstly, no amount of working out or eating can make a human being change their genetic body composition. What do I mean by this? Simply put, if you are an ectomorph, that's a term that is used to describe someone who is essentially skinny and is unable to put on significant muscle mass, then even with proper exercising and great eating you won't be able to change that much. Again, I'm not in the business of lying to anyone or putting out nonsense. There're a ton of books out there selling false dreams however I will never do this. I have a reputation of telling it like it is. This does not mean that you cannot maximize what you have. You can certainly improve whatever base you have through a logical workout plan and a healthy meal plan. However, when you see those ads or posts on social media with people saying that they have gained forty pounds of muscle in six months or a year that is complete baloney. I'll put it this way, I was 180lbs when I graduated high school and I'm still 180lbs at 29 years old. I've been working out and eating healthy since I was around eleven years old. As you can see I'm not just saying this stuff. I'm living proof of this theory. Now some of you may say, well maybe you are different. Perhaps I am incapable of changing much and I am unique in that way. Perhaps some people can drastically change. I'm only telling you my personal observations. You should look up Herschel Walker and you will see that he was the same size in high school and college as he is now over thirty years later.

Those people who drastically change are usually cheating by using sports enhancement drugs such as steroids and growth hormone. I have been in the sports world most of my life and I can tell you that illegal drug use is rampant. Moreover, when it comes to bodybuilding it is commonplace. Therefore, I'm here to tell you to be realistic with your expectations. Love yourself. Don't try to be something that you are not or try to be something that requires putting your health at risk. Everything in life has a consequence. Sometimes the consequence happens quickly; sometimes it takes a long time. Trust me when I tell you that I have seen some horror stories of people who have used steroids, especially when I worked in the hospital. Now that that is out of the way let me reveal the reason for discussing that topic first.

Training one muscle group is a waste of time. Why? For the very reason that I stated above, this is propagated by gym meatheads that say something like, "bro, we gonna go hard on chest today, big chest bro, only chest." Well, those same guys may or may not be heavily muscled however they are probably heavily muscled due to exogenous hormone use, i.e. steroids. Whether you train one body part per day or four body parts per day, you will likely stay around the same size naturally. However, training multiple body parts per day will keep you leaner, save you time, and keep the workout more interesting.

Thus, training multiple body parts each day is just better, put simply. I was once a teenager and I tried the ridiculous one body part a day. As I said before, it won't yield the best results because you won't be burning as many calories. Additionally, as you will learn, waiting a whole six or seven days to train the same body part again is also a big waste of time and overkill. Depending of course on the individual, most people, granted they have sufficient diets, will heal a muscle group anywhere from 48 hours to 72 hours post workout. Only if you are a beginner do you need more time for recovery.

Another benefit of training multiple body parts each day is the fact that if I ever do miss a workout I have that covered as I can just roll in my missed muscle groups on the next workout or I can literally just miss that day altogether since I train each muscle group so often each week.

Here's a funny misconception that I hear all the time when people learn that I train so many body parts per workout. They often say that I would be bigger if I trained one body part instead. Sorry my female readers who are probably grimacing at this section of the book however yes, males do talk about this type of nonsense. Men are biologically programmed to want to be alpha and bigger often registers as more alpha for men. Now back to the misconception; no, I would likely not be bigger as I discussed above. Secondly, who really cares about being a huge monstrous man? I find this strange and a direct reflection of our current obsessions with extremes.

Alternatively, on the female side of things, I've also seen women who are obsessed with a certain extreme aesthetic. Let me be the voice of reason for you all and tell you that you are beautiful the way that you are and you do not need to be so extreme. Just be healthy and be the best that you can be in a healthy way. The number one way to know that you are achieving the best version of yourself is your health. If your health is being compromised then that means that you are not doing things the right way. With optimal health comes maximum performance as well.

I understand of course that this section is about training multiple body parts each workout however, if I don't add value through advice I would feel as if I'm doing you, the reader, a disservice. A lot of the topics that I discuss most people avoid or don't want to confront.

In conclusion, I think that you can understand the benefits of training multiple body parts every workout. You can also understand the logic behind doing it this way. For those of you have never tried working out multiple muscle groups every workout, I encourage you to give it a shot. I bet that you're going to like it. If you have no idea where to begin, just use my workout in the previous chapter as a starting point. Remember to listen to your body, be smart, and in tune with it. You will most likely need to craft your own perfect workout for your body as I did for myself. Don't think that my workout is the best workout for every single person. Regarding women, a lot of you definitely do not have my goals when it comes to the way you want to look. Thus, you will likely not utilize my workout and that's fine. However, you should do some form of weight training because of bone composition and skeletal muscle. Women lose bone density past the age of thirty at a consistent rate as well as skeletal muscle. It's important for you to do weight bearing exercises. If you do not want to bulk up, do circuit type workouts that are fast paced and high intensity.

Why is cardio so important?

Cardio is the most important part of your workout. Every single human being should do at least 15 minutes of cardio 5 days a week. That's so ridiculously easy to accomplish. We all have at least 15 minutes of spare time. You can literally go in your living room and run in place for 15 minutes and there you go. Okay, so why is cardio so important?

Before we get into that, let me tell you how I personally discovered the importance of cardio. As a kid I played sports. I played soccer, I ran track, I played football, and I played basketball. I even tried swimming. Thus, cardio was always a big part of my life. When I started weight training seriously around freshman year of college I hardly did any cardio. I thought, "Why do it" since I read as many people do that weight training is enough. Well that is just not the case. During the end of my undergraduate academic college career I decided to join the Columbia soccer team.

Thus, I began doing cardio again. After a couple of years of no cardio and only weight training I was out of breath almost immediately. Moreover I just didn't feel the way that I once did. It was a very strange feeling and experience when you could no longer do what you once did. The bottom line is that I was out of shape.

Fast forward after several intense and grueling weeks of nonstop cardio training I was slowly returning back to form in terms of feeling better. Surprisingly, I noticed some added benefits, even though I was doing a ton of cardio, my body actually started to look like I was getting more muscular and I was getting stronger in the gym. All of my lifts were going up.

This was very surprising to me because literally everyone that I knew from the gym world told me that I'm going to lose all of my muscle and all of my strength from all of the cardio. They couldn't have been more wrong. If you lift weights, do cardio, and eat a proper diet you will likely improve in every category. All of the false information saying that cardio will remove your hard earned muscle or results is just nonsense. Okay, so that is my experience. Now let's get into the science.

Why is cardio so great scientifically speaking and what is actually happening on a bio-physiological level?

Cardio improves your cardiovascular health. Aerobic exercise, not anaerobic, is the only way to strengthen your heart. Cardio helps your heart pump blood more efficiently throughout your body. Cardiovascular exercise has also been shown to help lower blood pressure, that's why athletes that run a lot almost always have a very low resting blood pressure and heart rate. Their hearts don't have to work very hard at rest. Cardio keeps arteries clear through cholesterol metabolism, essentially raising "good" high-density lipoprotein (HDL) cholesterol and lowering "bad" low-density lipoprotein (LDL). Here's a cool trick that I used in undergrad as well as in medical school to remember what was good cholesterol and what was bad cholesterol. Always remember protein is good and protein is heavier than fat per same volume, thus protein is higher density. High-density lipoprotein cholesterol is such called HDL because it contains a much higher percentage of protein than LDL. Hopefully that helps you keep that straight.

Cardio helps regulate your blood sugar. With exercise insulin levels are regulated and with insulin regulation blood sugar is often kept lower. Too much sugar in your blood is referred to in the medical field as "sticky blood" which makes complete sense because if you pour table sugar into a small container of water you will see how it gets gelatin like and very sticky. That's especially dangerous for your cardiovascular system. This is why so many people suffer from cardiovascular problems: diet, lack of exercise, and too much sugar in the diet. There have been numerous studies which you can Google because I don't feel like citing them here and they're all over the place that show how cardiovascular exercise lowers the risk of type 2 diabetes as well as helps people with type 2 diabetes with management, even sometimes reversing the type 2 diabetes altogether.

Cardio also reduces asthma symptoms. If you have asthma like I did as a kid, ironically, cardio will help lessen both the frequency and severity of your asthma attacks. However, please consult your doctor if you do indeed have asthma as everyone's case is different and he or she may have specific precautions or may recommend specific activities. Nonetheless, my asthma definitely abated as I did more cardio when I was a kid.

These days so many people have chronic back pain, especially from sitting in a computer chair all day and then commuting back and forth from work sitting in your car seat. No matter how comfortable your work chair and car seat are, it is not healthy to sit down for a long duration of time. I encourage you to always think about why I'm saying what I'm saying. Here's why I know that sitting is not healthy or natural. Think about how we evolved as human beings. Were we sitting down on chairs or seats? No, we were not. We evolved in such a way that sitting in a chair is in fact unnatural for us. When it comes to health you will see that my philosophies are deeply routed in evolutionary biology and science. When I think about optimal diet and exercise I think about how we evolved. It's like trying to optimize the health of a lion. Lions are predators that eat meat and hunt. Therefore, it wouldn't be logical to feed a lion a vegetarian diet and have the lion in a pond. The lion wouldn't likely live very long. Now for vegetarians reading this, don't take that personal, I'm not comparing you to a lion. Vegetarian diets are great if you know what you're doing and if they work for your body type and genetics. With my genetic makeup and the region of the world that my ancestors come from a vegetarian diet would not be good. My ancestors lived off of milk, cheese, and meat for hundreds of years. You need to always think about where you came from when considering your ideal diet and exercise plan. Now back to cardio.

Another great benefit of cardio is that it helps you sleep better. I read several studies about individuals that had chronic sleep issues. A group of these people were selected to engage in regular cardiovascular exercise and positive results were demonstrated. For someone like me who doesn't sleep much cardio is essential. Tip: exercising too close to bedtime can make it difficult to sleep, I recommend giving yourself two hours between the end of your workout and when you go to sleep if you workout in the evening.

This is an obvious one, but cardio of course regulates your weight. I for one will get way to big (in a bad way) if I don't do cardio. I need to maintain low calories and I absolutely need to do cardio, especially as I get older. I do only 15 minutes of cardio 5 to 6 days a week and because I am consistent with cardio as well as my diet I am able to maintain a low body fat. I'm not special. You can do this too. I encourage you to research studies on how cardio alone helped people lose significant weight and by keeping up with the cardio these people were able to maintain their weight loss. I always believe that your diet should be optimized but some of those studies had people that didn't even change their diets, yet they still lost weight. A good cardio session can help you burn anywhere from 400 to 600 calories, now this is all dependent on how long you do your cardio for as well as the intensity. I usually burn a little less than 200 calories according to the machine during my 15 minutes. Again, remember that these machines are not designed specifically for you. There's no way we can assess how many calories any one person burns per time interval during any form of exercise because everyone has different levels of efficiencies within their metabolic pathways and different levels of efficiencies in their energy consumption. I'm not going to get deep into the science here but look out for another book and I will take you through all of the metabolic pathways from literally ingesting a food stuff to producing ATP.

Cardio strengthens your immune system. It has been shown that regular and moderate aerobic exercise will increase antibodies in the blood, these are called immunoglobulins. Increased amount of immunoglobulins means a stronger immune system to fight off pathogens such as viruses, bacteria, and fungi.

Regular cardio will lower your cortisol levels. I'm sure that you've heard of cortisol. It really is as bad as it is made out to be. High cortisol levels have such a wide spectrum of negative health effects that I could write a book on just that. However, in a nutshell, high cortisol, the stress hormone, will make you more tired, make you gain weight, and contribute to depression. Therefore, do your cardio!

Cardio has been shown to improve your brainpower. You may not know this and this is pretty depressing but it has been shown that just like it is a fact that women lose bone density after 30 years old, we all start losing brain tissue after 30 as well. This means that our cognitive abilities may start to lower. However, cardio has been shown to slow down this process. How did scientists analyze this? They used magnetic resonance imaging (MRI) scans to evaluate older adults with a wide range of health and aerobic fitness levels and they saw that the more fit adults had larger amounts of brain tissue.

If you are ever down, go for a run. Cardio will boost your mood. We all get depressed from time to time. That's normal. Life is a sine wave, you'll probably hear me say that again as it's one of my favorite phrases. There're constant peaks and valleys in life. You have to understand this. Life is not easy. It is very hard. Prepare yourself for that reality and don't be delusional into thinking that your life will ever be all peaches and roses. I'm sorry to tell you but it won't be. You are human just like all of us. No human being is immune to the realities of living. Okay, so go for a run. Whenever I go for a run most of the things in my life get blocked out and even if they aren't necessarily blocked out I at least start to feel a boost in my mood. This is due to endorphins being released, so-called the runner's high.

For the elderly, cardio is even more important. The older you get the more important it is to workout and do cardio. Life is ironic like that. When we are young, strong, and full of life we take life for granted. A lot of us don't eat healthy and we don't exercise regularly. Many of us get away with that for a large portion of our youth without any severe ramifications. However, when you get older, everything catches up. There is always a reaction to your action. There is always an effect whether it happens now or in fifty years. For older adults, it is especially important to do cardio and even though this chapter is about cardio, I'm going to say, it's especially important for older adults to perform weight-bearing exercises. Many elderly people end up breaking bones due to falls, which is extremely common amongst people over the age of 65 with a reported incidence of one in every three people. A bad fall can leave a person permanently disabled. Therefore, if you are young get into the habit of doing cardio and exercising and if you are an older adult please try your best to build good habits. I'm rooting for you!

Three of the best things about cardiovascular exercise are it is safe, affordable, and accessible. Cardio is usually safe for most people and you have so much flexibility regarding what type of cardio you can do. Cardio is also super cheap; you literally don't need any equipment or a gym membership to do cardio. Moreover, you can do cardio anywhere.

In conclusion, I hope that I presented to you why cardio is so important and I convinced you if you don't already do cardio to give it a shot. I think you will be thanking me later on, and more importantly, you will be thanking yourself for doing it.

The Career Diet

Now things get really interesting and as some say, "really good" because I'm going to teach you how to eat relatively stress free for the remainder of your life. Before we get into the explanation, let me give you some advice that you may or may not know by now. Please don't stress about anything that you cannot control anymore. I did this for most of my life until one day I realized that all of the things that I'm stressing about are out of my hands. You cannot control what other people are going to do. You can't control the weather. You can't control the economy. There're very few things that you can control in this world. Fortunately, diet is one of them!

Ironically, the career diet is pretty much the type of diet I'd recommend for anyone really. The entire fitness industry promotes extremely strict eating, primarily with scheduling and multiple meals a day. This is 100% wrong. In fact, it will likely hurt you more than help you. How do I know? Well I of course tried out virtually every diet out there and I happen to be a biochemist that specializes in metabolism. Now one thing I want to point out is that just because someone understands the science and theory behind something does not necessarily mean that that person is an expert. When I was in medical school, everyone in my class was extremely intelligent and understood metabolic pathways to a pretty high level. However, most of my colleagues did not understand how to eat properly or workout effectively. Some did. Therefore, what I'm trying to say is you need application to really become an expert in an area and more than anything else you need to see results. Perhaps a big reason why you're reading this book is because you have seen that I do practice what I preach and I do in fact have the results to show for what I'm saying.

Now, why are there so many diets out there and why are there so many complicated diets? It's very simple: money, money, and more money. This world revolves around money and everyone is looking how to make the next buck. Today the hottest diet plan says we need to eat eight times a day 2oz of chicken each time to speed up our metabolism and take this shake in between and tomorrow it's five times a day only fish along with a veggie smoothie. I'm just giving you examples here. Diet plans are fads. I'm not offering you any fad diet. I'm giving you the diet that you should stick to for the rest of your life.

So, how should the diet look? As with all things, the diet must be logical. The diet plan that I recommend follows simple rules that I will get into. But the main thing is that there really isn't any set time to eat other than breakfast. So here are the rules:

1. You must eat breakfast, when I was in medical school I had to skip breakfast often, and this had negative effects on me. If you are in a huge rush in the morning I will provide a solution for you.
2. You only need three to four meals a day maximum.
3. You must eat your carbs early on in the day.
4. You must have the proper balance of carbs, proteins, and fats.
5. You need to drink water throughout the day.
6. You need to eat veggies.
7. You need to eat fruit.
8. You should never take any supplements of any kind unless doctor recommended. I do not take any supplements. That means I do not take any protein powder or anything that you can purchase at GNC or a health food store. These products are low grade and not regulated. When I had my organic food company, the number one reason we formed the company, was to provide people with real food on the go. Our products had only four ingredients inside and no preservatives and nothing artificial. Unfortunately, when I went away to medical school we sold the company, as I couldn't do both. In any case, I will give you easy solutions for quick meals.
9. You should always eat healthy fats at night.
10. You should not cut out your salt if you workout.

Okay, so those are some general rules you should follow moving forward. Now let's take a look at what a typical day should look like regarding the diet and let's dissect each element.

The following will outline an entire day for a busy professional; let's call her Carla. Carla wakes up at 6:00AM. She takes a quick shower and heads to the kitchen. She's always in a rush because she needs to be at work at 9:00AM and beat the traffic. So Carla is in the kitchen. Everything is already organized because if you're kitchen is not organized you're going to have major issues being efficient. Carla gets a large bowl and grabs the oatmeal. She puts the bowl on a scale and tares the scale. You need to purchase a scale. Trust me, this will help tremendously. There are two types of people; People who under-eat like me and people who overeat. I personally always eat less than the amount I should unless I weigh my food. Weighing your food will keep you in check. Also since we are on the weighing topic. You should weigh yourself every morning so that you can keep data points. The more data points you can have the more objective you can be about yourself and your life. So Carla now weighs out 40 grams of oatmeal into the bowl.

Next Carla grabs cocoa powder, flax powder, and ground chia seeds. She puts all three inside with the oatmeal. I don't weigh these ingredients. If you want to weigh them I'd say 20 grams of each works well. Next Carla grabs cloves and nutmeg and sprinkles a little bit of each on her oatmeal. The final step before putting the oatmeal in the microwave is to go and get one or two whole eggs, crack them, and put them in. Add water and mix everything up before putting everything in the microwave for 2 minutes.

As the oatmeal is being made, Carla uses this time to pack a lunch for herself of premade chicken and broccoli. Always prepare enough chicken or fish for two to three days. This way you always have healthy food available. Carla weighs her chicken of course – 4 oz. and as much broccoli as she desires. Now Carla is done packing her lunch and her oatmeal is also ready.

She takes her warm chocolate flavored oatmeal out and adds in organic whole milk yogurt. Organic whole milk yogurt is one of the best probiotic rich foods and will keep your digestive system healthy. Next she chooses her fruit. She likes pineapple, it's already cut, and she adds it in with a tablespoon of honey. You should eat local honey because honey will help your immune system get used to local allergens. I learned this trick when I was in my late teens as I had horrible allergies. I always look for natural ways to improve health. Don't overeat fruit. Believe it or not too much fruit can make you fat. At least, I know with my genetics I can definitely get fat from eating too much fruit. You need to be realistic about your body type. I hear people all the time that are delusional about their respective body types. If you really want to know your body type just look at your parents and the rest of your family.

I come from a region of the world where people don't have access to a lot of food. Therefore, if I eat even 2000 calories I gain weight and put on size, which is not my personal goal. Thus, I need to keep my calories in the neighborhood of about 1200-1500. Everybody is different. However, I recommend always keeping your calories low for health reasons. It's been shown through many research articles that low calorie and low carb diets prolong life. Too much food will overtax your organs and your body will work very hard on breaking everything down.

Okay, so that's pretty much breakfast. You can also add in some almond butter with your oatmeal if you like. However, I don't do this. Since I exercise really hard with weights I sometimes will eat chicken and broccoli along with my oatmeal so that I can have a big breakfast as once my work day starts I often don't eat for many hours later. In any case, only do what I do if you exercise intensely with weights and you want to keep muscle mass. For most people, this would be unnecessary and probably not desired.

Now it is several hours later and Carla's lunchtime has arrived. Since Carla has packed her food she has no stress of what to eat and there is no risk that she may eat poorly. The number one reason that I have witnessed that people stray from a healthy diet is because most people don't pack their lunches and they end up eating out. Most food from outside is not healthy, even the food that is promoted as health food. To be your best you really should try to pack your food and of course cook all your food. For those of you that don't know how to cook, it's super easy. Just watch some tutorials on YouTube.

Here's a cook summary of how to cook chicken. Preheat your oven to 375 degrees Fahrenheit. I personally like chicken thighs. Put two to three days worth of chicken thighs in a tray or two. I use metal cooking trays made with metals that have melting points that don't put me at risk for any metal deposition in my food. You should do the same. Once the chicken is in the tray, I add garlic, oregano, salt, pepper, parsley, onion, and basil. All of these spices can be purchased at Wholefoods or any food store. Very important: try to eat organic everything. Since you don't need to eat a ton of food, eat organic. The cost difference will be minimal. And yes, even for my friends who are reading this and are bodybuilders, you don't need to eat 8 meals a day and if you do eat 8 meals a day you're probably not going to be very good at your job or career and you will also likely have health problems later on in life, specifically with your kidneys. Take it from me, you can easily Google me and see that I have maintained my muscle mass with anywhere from 2 to 4 meals per day, and small meals. I'm not special. The muscle mass is a direct correlation of how hard you train and genetics. I was the same weight that I am now when I was a teenager and about the same strength. Those who think that you're going to change dramatically will learn that you can't believe everything you read in muscle magazines or see on television. People that you see have radical changes are on steroids, plain and simple. Also, whenever I say that I'm going to put on size or get bigger I am talking about increased body fat. I don't think I can add more muscle mass than I already have on my frame.

Therefore, I encourage you to devote your energy to more meaningful things than eating 8 times a day. You can accomplish so much more by just eating 3 or 4 meals per day and not following such a strict program. That's my advice for people who are obsessed with bodybuilding and fitness. As I always say, ironically, the person who eats 3 or 4 meals will probably look better than the person who eats 8 meals because it's very unhealthy to overload your body with so much excess food.

Thus, as a career professional you should never feel like you are missing out because you can't follow these diets that you see posted on the web. So far Carla has had breakfast and her lunch. Her lunch consisted of 4 oz. of chicken and broccoli. She has also been drinking water throughout the morning and early afternoon. It's a good habit to drink one glass of water before eating and one glass after eating. Try to keep water bottles with you at all times. This way you can always be hydrated.

Now you may be wondering when did Carla eat lunch? Remember when I said, that you need to be flexible. It doesn't matter when she ate lunch. You can eat lunch at noon or you can eat lunch at 3PM. As long as you eat lunch that's what's important and most importantly, lunch must be healthy. Don't put pressure on yourself that you need to eat at some pre-designated time. That is complete nonsense. Your goal is to be good at your career and adding value to the world. Eating healthy and exercising should only complement this overall life mission and aid in your pursuits.

Carla's day is coming to a close. She drives to the gym to do a quick one-hour workout as discussed previously. After her workout she comes home and eats dinner. Now some of you are probably wondering, do you need to eat something before you workout? It all depends, for some yes, for some no. For me, I will eat the same meal that I had for lunch before I go the gym, thus, I'll have a third meal, however this isn't required and often times when I was in medical school I wouldn't do this. Honestly, for guys who lift heavy like me having a little bit more protein and veggies before the workout helps. I also eat around 6-8 oz. of chicken instead of 4 oz. Women should not eat more than 4 oz. I will provide a sample diet plan at the end of the book for you guys.

So what does Carla eat for dinner? Dinner is like breakfast, it's vital and it's unique. So far if you've noticed, we only eat carbohydrates for breakfast. If you want to be lean for the rest of your life this is what you must do; carbs only in the morning. For dinner, we eat protein and fats. Carla will eat 4 oz. of chicken or fish with some type of green vegetable that does not have sugar such as broccoli, asparagus, or spinach. She will also have a healthy fat source of her choosing. You can eat avocado, almond butter, cheese (if you are not lactose intolerant), or cashew butter. Those are my top fat choices. Remember to drink water. Don't drink too much water or else you'll have to get up when you're sleeping to use the rest room.

Notice that I did not give you a specific time for when Carla ate dinner because that is irrelevant. Just eat dinner when you can eat dinner and be sure it's healthy. Do you see how easy this can be? It can even make your life more efficient if you do it correctly. Instead of pondering what restaurant or fast food place you're going to go order from you already have all the answers. I really hope that you can adapt to this because I know it will be so great for your life and bring you a lot of happiness. Looking and feeling your best always helps boost your mood. I hope that this was helpful and I hope that it shed light on how you should eat and how you should think about food as a busy career professional.

Before we conclude this chapter, if for whatever reason you do not have time to eat breakfast you will need to eat breakfast for lunch at work and then eat another meal before you go to the gym. That's the simple solution.

Why other diets fail for most people?

Most diets fail simply because they are fad diets that are unrealistic and too extreme. A no carb diet is unhealthy just like a no fat diet is unhealthy. My diet contains balance. You have carbs, fats, proteins, and all of the vitamins and nutrients that your body will need. It's interesting when you get on a fad diet. Yes, as I mentioned previously I've tried almost every diet out there. When I would get on one of these diets my body never felt right. That's how you know something is wrong. You need to try your best to listen to your body and trust your instincts. Your mind and body will literally tell you if something is off. If you eliminate carbohydrates completely from your diet guess what, your body will stop producing certain enzymes and the moment you do reintroduce carbohydrates back into your diet your body will no longer be efficient in breaking them down. In order for your body to up-regulate your enzyme production, it will need weeks, sometimes, months and years to get back to normal levels. This is why fad diets don't work. I don't think there's much more to say on the topic. Simply put most other diets don't work because they are unsustainable. My diet protocol may not be realistic for you either, you're the judge of that, and I'm just telling you the facts. If you want to look your best, be your healthiest, and live longer you should think about following my diet long-term.

Adapting your diet to any environment

Here is probably the most critical thing for you since you may travel for work or you may just be in situations where you can't pack your food. You already know what you can and can't eat. Thus, all it takes is a little bit of effort and you should always be able to find a solution. I traveled throughout the United States on many occasions for weeks at a time. I always found ways to eat properly and ways to exercise. Let's talk about eating healthily.

Wherever you are in the world you know what you need to eat for breakfast, lunch, and dinner. You know that you need to have your carbs and fruit in the morning. You know that you need your protein and veggies for lunch and you know that you need your protein, veggies and fats for dinner. Thus, it's so simple.

Let's use one of my real world experiences as an example. Back when I applied to medical school, I received interview invitations all over the country. Let's talk about the University of Missouri School of Medicine as this is an interesting place to discuss since it's in a rural place and Brad Pitt went to Mizzou for undergrad, pretty cool, that's the only fun fact I know about the place, oh and they party hard, but that's a topic for another book.

My interview was sometime in fall before Halloween. I made sure that I ate before my flight and since the flight was not going to be very long I didn't worry about food until after I got off the plane. Unfortunately, I had to connect, I want to say in Chicago, but I'm not 100 percent sure. Regardless, the flight got delayed. Most people would stress, especially considering the interview was at 8AM and I was going to get to Missouri after 12PM because of the delay. However, as I always tell you, don't stress about things you can't control. Thus, I was pretty relaxed and I just adjusted.

I already had my breakfast and a lunch. All I needed was a healthy dinner so that I can be at maximum performance for my interview. I'm used to not getting much sleep. Thus, I wasn't concerned. I can always pull at least one all-nighter and maintain about 90 percent or so of my mental and physical abilities since I'm used to that. This is a topic for another book but once upon a time I needed to work two jobs and go to school at the same time. I also made time to workout, calisthenics. Thus, those few years conditioned me for working hard with little sleep and ever since I've been able to adapt to such conditions. For me, food intake is probably more important than sleep. Okay, so my only shot at eating dinner was the airport.

I looked around and I found a place that looked like a chipotle. As I said before, food from outside is never ideal but in situations like this it's going to have to do. Thus, I went and ordered a bowl consisting of chicken, veggies, and avocado. My healthy meal was a success. The moral of the story is where there is a will there is a way. Don't let yourself deviate from plans due to excuses that you create for yourself. Try not to waiver on your values. Committing yourself to eating healthily and exercising is an expression of your values. That's my opinion. Just like you always get work done no matter what. Get the food and exercise done for you as well.

Just like you adapted with the diet, you can also adapt with the exercise routine. Research where there will be gyms. Book your hotel near one. If you have no gym, do calisthenics and cardio every day.

How to stick to the plan

The number one way to stick to any plan is to start NOW! Seriously, don't wait for tomorrow. Don't wait for the New Year. Don't wait for some external factor to propel you to begin your plan. If you rely on anything but an internal force that comes from deep within yourself you're going to fail – trust me, I've seen this time and time again in many facets of life, not just dieting and exercising. The only way that any person can change is if that individual wants to change. It's not about whether someone else wants that person to change. Additionally, if the reason you are making a change is for another person, thing, or anything other than you, it is highly unlikely the change will stick. You may have witnessed this harsh reality yourself in life or you may have not. For those who are older and more experienced I'm sure you know what I'm talking about. For those of you who are younger, there's not much I can say about this topic as everyone is going to live their own lives. I just hope you don't make the same mistakes that I made and try to do anything for superficial reasons or worse try to change anyone else who doesn't want to change even if those changes are wholeheartedly for the betterment of that person.

So sticking to the plan is simple. Begin immediately. Keep track of everything. Build your good habits. Hold yourself accountable. Watch motivational videos. In fact, as I say in my books, I encourage you to always watch motivational videos and surround yourself with things that will build you up, inspire you, and push you to be better. You are the average of those around you. There's a saying like that. It's very true. There were times in my life when I needed to isolate myself from most of the people around me because I recognized that those people were not positive people. Thus, I did exactly what I'm telling you to do – I watched motivational videos, I read inspirational books, I became friends with some of the greatest minds that walked the planet: Plato, Socrates, Rousseau, Michelangelo, Einstein, Newton, and many others. If you immerse yourself in greatness you will become better and better. You may never become as great as those people aforementioned, I certainly never will, but the most important thing is that you are the best version of yourself.

Here are some practical tips for sticking to your plan. First and foremost, write out a detailed concrete plan that you will stick to. Write out what you're going to do and the steps. For instance, you need to go food shopping. Right out a list of all of the food items you will need. Next write out how your diet will look. This should be easy since I'm going to write out a diet here for you. Write out a workout plan. I included how to workout in a previous chapter. Use that as a guideline. Join a gym. You know what I did when I first started working out? I literally had my favorite motivational video on repeat and I would watch it several times whenever I was free. That way I was pumped up to go to the gym. That works. Download good music. Invest in some Bluetooth headphones. Go buy some new workout gear. All of these things will get you in the mood.

As for sticking to your diet, there's no easy way to say this but it's not going to be easy. I purposely wrote a double easy if you're wondering. Sticking to my diet won't be easy. I realize that. Unfortunately, you know another favorite thing I say, nothing worth having is easy. Seriously, if you acquired something with ease, 9 out 10 times it's something that is not worth it; it's something anybody can have. The same goes for your health and for your body.

Remember the laws of thermodynamics and more importantly the law of entropy. We are in a constant state of decay. The universe is constantly becoming more and more disordered. The same is true for us. We need to put a tremendous amount of focus and energy into preserving ourselves for the long term. It requires discipline, tenacity, and a strong mind. The mind is the most important part of anything that you will ever do.

Bonus: diet

Meal 1
40 grams of oatmeal (dry old fashioned steel cut) made with water
½ cup strawberries
6 egg whites cooked with 1 yolk (male)
3 egg whites cooked with 1 yolk (female)

Meal 2
1 cup green vegetables (best options are broccoli, asparagus, and brussel sprouts)
6-8 oz. chicken breast (grilled and no sauce) (male)
4 oz. chicken breast (female)

Meal 3
Tuna salad made with 8 oz. tuna (in oil or water), 4 Tbsp. mayonnaise (male)
Tuna salad made with 4 oz. tuna (in oil or water), 4 Tbsp. mayonnaise (female)
1 Tbsp. almond butter
1 cup green vegetables

For a great book on how to start out your journey please check out my book "Lean in 30 Days" on Amazon.